# *Alkaline Smoothies*

---

*Reset Your Metabolism with Healthy and Easy Smoothie Recipes for Natural Weight Loss*

*Tiffany Aniston*

©Copyright 2021 – *Tiffany Aniston* - All rights reserved

The content contained within this book may not be reproduced, duplicated, or transmitted without direct written permission from the author or the publisher.

Under no circumstances will any blame or legal responsibility be held against the publisher, or author, for any damages, reparation, or monetary loss due to the information contained within this book, either directly or indirectly.

Legal Notice

This book is copyright protected. This book is only for personal use. You cannot amend, distribute, sell, use, quote or paraphrase any part, or the content within this book, without the consent of the author-publisher.

Disclaimer Notice

Please note the information contained within this document is for educational and entertainment purposes only. All effort has been executed to present accurate, up to date, and reliable, complete information. No warranties of any kind are declared or implied. Readers acknowledge that the author is not engaging in the rendering of legal, financial, medical, or professional advice.

# Table of Contents

**Introduction** ............................................................................................. 6

**Chapter 1:** *Understanding the Meaning of Alkaline* ................... 7

    The Importance of a balanced pH in the body............................. 8

    Health Problems Due to Acidity in the Body ............................... 8

    Why Fruit Vegetable Smoothies Maintain a Proper pH .............. 9

    Healthy Eating Guidelines for Preventing Cancer .................... 11

**Chapter 2:** *Best Alkaline Foods* ............................................... 13

**Chapter 3:** *What You Need to Get Started* ............................... 20

    Getting Started as a Beginner .................................................. 20

    How to Make a Good, Natural Smoothie.................................. 20

    How to Get the Right Herbs ..................................................... 22

    What to Expect During the Smoothie Detox? .......................... 22

    Tips to Motivate You to Get Started ......................................... 24

**Chapter 4: Smoothies Recipes** .................................................. 26

    1. Avocado Blueberry Smoothie ............................................. 26

    2. Veggie-Ful Smoothie .......................................................... 27

    3. Detox Sugar Smoothie ....................................................... 28

    4. Walnut Milk and Dandelion Smoothie .............................. 29

    5. Blueberry Pie Smoothie ..................................................... 30

    6. Lettuce, Blueberry, and Coconut Smoothie ...................... 31

    7. Kale Banana Smoothie ...................................................... 32

    8. Vanilla Spinach, Banana, Grape and Apple Smoothie ..... 33

    9. Ginger Avocado, Apple, Carrot, Kale Smoothie ............... 34

    10. Spinach Peanut Butter Smoothie ..................................... 35

    11. Rhubarb, Banana, Cranberry Smoothie........................... 36

    12. Cinnamon Apple, Pear, Spinach Smoothie...................... 37

    13. Honeydew, Grapes, Cucumber, Broccoli Smoothie......... 38

14. Minty Melon Smoothie ................................................................. 39
15. Orange Banana Green Smoothie ............................................... 40
16. Orange Zucchini Smoothie ........................................................ 41
17. Fruity Herbal Tea Smoothie ...................................................... 42
18. Cucumber Smoothie .................................................................. 43
19. Swiss Chard Smoothie ............................................................... 44
20. Mint Smoothie ........................................................................... 45
21. Zucchini and Dill Smoothie ...................................................... 46
22. Kiwi and Lemon Smoothie ....................................................... 47
23. Apple, Walnut, and Green Smoothie ....................................... 48
24. Pineapple Coconut Detox Smoothie ........................................ 49
25. Avocado Detox Smoothie ......................................................... 50
26. Chamomile Ginger Detox Smoothie ........................................ 51
27. Wheatgrass Detox Smoothie .................................................... 52
28. Charcoal Lemonade Detox Smoothie ...................................... 53
29. Banana Oatmeal Detox Smoothie ............................................ 54
30. Apple Chia Detox Smoothie ..................................................... 55
31. Dandelion Greens and Mixed Berry Smoothie ....................... 56
32. Baby Spinach and Pear Smoothie ............................................ 57
33. Spicy Spinach Smoothie ........................................................... 59
34. Romaine Lettuce and Ginger Smoothie .................................. 60
35. Peach Yogurt Smoothie ............................................................ 61
36. Creamy Carrot Smoothie .......................................................... 62
37. Blackberry Apple Smoothie ..................................................... 63
38. Fruit Medley Smoothie ............................................................. 64
39. Papaya and Quinoa Smoothie .................................................. 65
40. Choco Collards ........................................................................... 66
41. Peach Green Smoothie .............................................................. 67
42. Choy Choco ................................................................................ 68

| | | |
|---|---|---|
| 43. | Parsley with Mixed Cherry Smoothie | 69 |
| 44. | Apple Berry Green Smoothie | 70 |
| 45. | Strawberry Banana Green Smoothie | 71 |
| 46. | Maple, Banana, Kale Smoothie | 72 |
| 47. | Tropical Kiwi Green Smoothie | 73 |
| 48. | Tropical Green Kiwi Smoothie II | 74 |
| 49. | Celery with Orange Smoothie | 75 |
| 50. | Swiss Chard Jazz | 76 |
| 51. | Dandelion with Mango | 77 |
| 52. | Sprouts Sizzles | 78 |
| 53. | Honey Green Veg | 79 |
| 54. | Romaine Lettuce with Peach and Avocado | 80 |
| 55. | Pain-Reducing Pineapple Ginger | 81 |
| 56. | Blueberry Basil Anti-Inflammatory | 82 |
| 57. | Papaya Coconut Inflammation Fighter | 83 |
| 58. | Cherry Rooibos | 84 |
| 59. | Coconut Carrot | 85 |
| 60. | Pineapple Cherry Pain Fighter | 86 |
| 61. | Celery and Beet Juice | 87 |
| 62. | Green Almond Milk Smoothie | 88 |
| 63. | Green Citrus Juice | 89 |
| 64. | Cold Fighting Green Smoothie | 90 |
| 65. | Fruit and Vegetable Cocktail | 91 |
| 66. | Kiwi Mint Smoothie | 92 |
| 67. | Avocado Smoothie | 93 |
| 68. | Green Lemonade | 94 |
| 69. | Sweet Spinach Detox | 95 |
| 70. | Celery Blueberry Smoothie | 96 |

**Conclusion** .................................................................................. **97**

# Introduction

The human body is alkaline in structure. By keeping it in the right ratio, it will run at the perfect level. Too much or insufficient alkaline will disturb the body's balance. Acidosis is created after some time.

Acidosis will cripple our body's basic functions without therapeutic treatment. Acidosis is a condition in which there is too much acid in body fluids. It is the opposite of alkalosis (a condition in which there is too much base in the body fluids). It makes our body exceptionally helpless against certain diseases, for example, diabetes, cancer, joint pain, just as heart diseases.

We must locate the correct method to diminish its creation. life. Among the recognized methods are exercise and a proper diet and a decrease in stress. A healthy way of life enables our body to keep its acid waste at the most reduced level possible.

The alkaline diet, otherwise called the pH wonder diet, appears to fit the structure of the human body. People who have specific health issues and need to limit certain foods will not fit it suitable.

# Chapter 1:
## *Understanding the Meaning of Alkaline*

The term, alkaline, refers to a substance that produces a neutral pH (or basic) when dissolved in water such as baking soda and potash. Alkaline are compounds have an alkaline ion H+ or OH-. As it turns out, many foods are either acidic or alkaline, depending upon what they contain and how the body breaks them down.

The scale of acidity or alkalinity is measured on a pH scale. Each number on the pH scale represents a factor of ten. For example, a solution that measures 3 is ten times more acid than a solution that measures 4. An acid will lower the pH of a solution. A base will raise the pH of a solution.

At room temperature, water is neutral; it doesn't change the volume of any object (water doesn't expand or contract). But all substances have different natures and react differently to different conditions. Water can be split into oxygen and hydrogen atoms, with an equal number of protons and electrons in each atom. This is called electrolysis, or an alkaline solution. An acid will release hydrogen ions (H+) and oxygen ions (. O2-) in water, which lowers the pH of a solution.

The discharge of H+ is related to the dissociation constant, which is the equilibrium constant for the reaction. The greater the value of the equilibrium constant, the greater the release of hydrogen ions in water. The most common way to measure this is by using a pH meter/pH indicator paper.

# The Importance of a balanced pH in the body

## Alkaline Blood and the Role of pH

Dr. Sebi's African Bio-Mineral Balance methodology introduced me to the concept that an acidic body supports the proliferation of disease, and an alkaline body protects against disease. The issue is a bit more complex, but for our purposes, it is true. More specifically, acidic blood supports the proliferation of disease.

Acid and alkaline are the opposite sides of the pH scale. The scale for pH ranges from 0pH to 14pH. 0pH represents the highest acidic level, and 14pH represents the highest alkaline level. 7.0pH is neutral. Although different areas of the body are acidic, it is very important to eat alkaline foods to maintain a blood pH of around 7.4. The pH of the blood is the reference point for homeostasis or optimal functioning of the organs in the body.

The body works diligently to keep the blood in a slightly alkaline state near a pH of 7.4 to support homeostasis and good health. pH stands for "potential hydrogen" and has the ability of molecules to attract hydrogen ions. Too many hydrogen ions in the bloodstream make the blood acidic and interferes with the proper oxygenation of cells. Eating meat, dairy, processed foods, and even highly hybridized, starchy plant foods acidify the blood because of their molecular structure. They also lack the vital minerals, vitamins, and phytonutrients the body needs to properly perform its metabolic functions.

## Health Problems Due to Acidity in the Body

Health problems due to acidity are becoming more and more

prevalent. Most people have begun to notice that they are suffering from many health-related problems such as blood pressure, headaches, depression, and heart disease. Studies show that the main cause of is the acidic nature of their bodies.

The intake of food is one way you can reduce your acidity levels. Foods like fruits, vegetables, legumes, and nuts can help lower your pH level as they have an alkalizing effect on the body. An overabundance of processed foods will have a different effect; therefore, it's important to reduce or stop eating these types of foods if you want to live a healthier life with less illness.

Another way to reduce acidity levels is by drinking alkaline water. It has been proven that adding magnesium to water can reduce the acidity in the body. When we eat certain food, many of the nutrients have an alkalizing effect on our body. It's recommended to drink ten glasses of water and one glass of fresh juice per day as these drinks will help keep your body alkaline. Alkaline foods such as cucumbers, green salads, and raw nuts can also be eaten to help you reach an alkaline pH level.

When ill, some people suffer from a highly acidic state. Pain relief, sleep, and relaxation can help you reduce the acidity in your body. Alkalize with herbs such as valerian root to help you fall asleep.

Alkaline foods also help you maintain a better mood. Try to eat more green vegetables such as spinach, lettuce, and celery because they are alkalizing and will give your body the minerals it needs to keep healthy. Water is a way for the body to excrete excess alkaline elements.

**Why Fruit Vegetable Smoothies Maintain a Proper pH**

Healthy eating is important, and the argument over which foods are healthiest is never-ending. There are many articles on the internet about healthy food, but few talk about fruit and vegetable smoothies. This book is devoted to the super food mixture.

Fruit is healthful because it contains a variety of nutrients like vitamins A, C, and E, potassium, fiber, and antioxidants to help protect cells from the damage caused by free radicals. It can be an effective tool for weight management because consuming whole fruits gives you a sense of fullness that prevents snacking on high-calorie foods like chocolate or cookies without the guilt often accompanying these indulgent foods.

The fiber in fruit also helps curb the appetite by encouraging the production of cholecystokinin, a hormone that causes the feeling of fullness. Whenever you eat fruits, cholecystokinin is released into your bloodstream, and this stimulates your brain to send a message to your stomach to tell it to stop eating.

The fiber in fruits also prevents nutritional deficiencies and constipation because it stimulates the production of a substance known as butyrate. Butyrate maintains normal intestinal function, relieves irregular bowel movements and thereby increases regularity.

It's a well-known fact that vegetables contain essential nutrients, such as calcium, potassium, and vitamins A, C, E, and K. Vegetables are also low in calories, so they can be consumed to boost metabolism and increase your energy level. They are incredibly good for the body because they can help relieve conditions like osteoporosis because they contain vitamin K, which helps reduce the risk of fractures by strengthening bones and teeth.

Vegetables are rich in antioxidants like beta-carotene and lutein that have been studied for their ability to protect against certain diseases, including age-related macular degeneration (AMD). AMD is a disease that can cause pain and vision loss in people over 65, and many studies have indicated that beta-carotene is shown to be very effective in preventing disease. In addition, lutein is a nutrient that helps maintain eye health because it promotes cell growth and prevents harmful free radicals from impairing vision or causing early blindness.

Finally, vegetables are very good for your body because they can reduce inflammation, reduce cholesterol and prevent cancer by slowing the growth of cells associated with certain cancers.

The bottom line is that fruit vegetable smoothies maintain a healthy pH and stimulate metabolism. They contain fiber to control appetite and promote regular bowel movements. Fiber is a powerful antioxidant helps prevent constipation and reduces high cholesterol.

**Healthy Eating Guidelines for Preventing Cancer**

The best way to ensure a healthy diet is to eat a variety of foods from all the major food groups every day. This can be done by including plenty of fresh fruits and vegetables in your meals. These foods are especially important because they contain powerful antioxidants, minerals, and vitamins that promote good health. It is a good idea to limit unhealthy fats, sugar, and salt by eating less processed foods and limiting consumption of foods high in fat, such as butter, cheese, and fatty meats. Avoiding or limiting the intake of sugary foods and drinks like sodas and pastries is also a good idea.

People concerned with their health should be especially mindful about keeping the sodium (salt) in their diet to a minimum because this substance has been linked to high blood pressure and other health problems. It is important to eat whole grains like brown rice, whole wheat bread, oatmeal, and quinoa because they lower the risk of heart disease by reducing LDL (bad) cholesterol levels in the body. Regular exercise that involves strength training along with daily physical activity will boost metabolism and strengthen muscles.

People even need to protect themselves against the health hazards of certain job. This is about exposure to strong chemical solvents, pesticides, ammonia, formaldehyde, and carbon monoxide. People who work with these chemicals should conduct an initial risk assessment to identify possible problems linked to exposure to chemical solvents and other dangerous substances.

Take precautions against exposure to these substances by using proper gloves, masks, or goggles when working with chemicals. (Of course, smoking can expose people to harmful toxins through their lungs.) Make certain that chemical storage areas are well-ventilated and kept at a safe distance from the workplace.

The best way to reduce exposure to potentially toxic products is to work in a well-ventilated area, don protective clothing, such as gloves or masks, and avoid touching your skin with chemical-soaked gloves or other materials.

# Chapter 2:
## *Best Alkaline Foods*

Almost all alkaline-forming foods can be considered as superfoods. It isn't just because of their ability to help the body keep a healthy pH balance but because of their nutrient density. Alkaline-forming foods are plant-based and have many healing properties.

You might know that it is very healthy to drink warm lime water or fresh green juice. They can improve the body's ability to detox, boost the immune system, and give you a huge dose of nutrients. All these can help raise the body's pH level, turning your system from being acid to alkaline.

If you were a good student during chemistry class, you might remember the concept of alkali versus acid. If you weren't, here is a refresher course. Acids will have a pH level less than seven, where alkalis will have a pH level of greater than seven. Water is the most neutral, with a pH of seven. Basically, this means that acids are corrosive in nature and sour in taste. Alkalis are used to neutralize acids.

When the body is in an alkaline state, it becomes more disease resistant, inhibiting the growth of organisms such as cancer, fungi, yeast, viruses, and bad bacteria. Oxygen levels get raised in our blood, organs, and tissues. This enables them to function more efficiently and effectively. It can reduce acidity and keep the alkaline state that encourages toxin excretion, energy production, and healthy cell turnover.

There are several factors that impact our body's pH levels. When we eat alkaline-forming foods and minimize how much acid-forming foods we consume, our bodies can keep up an alkaline state. An alkaline-forming food will be plant-based and rich in antioxidants, minerals, and vitamins. These are easier to digest and improve the gut's immune function, lowering mucus production and inflammation.

While our bodies are digesting, the stomach secretes gastric acid to break down the food. Our stomachs have a pH of between 2.0 and 3.5. This is very acidic, but we need it to be able to digest foods right. But there are times when because of bad food habits or bad lifestyle choices, the acid level goes haywire, causing gastric ailments, acid reflux, and other problems.

If you were to look at the normal diet of any American, it will contain huge amounts of acidic foods like pastries, doughnuts, colas, kebabs, bacon, sausages, cheese sandwiches, rolls, pizza, samosa, burgers, and many more that affect the acidic balance in our stomachs. When these foods get broken down, they leaves behind a residue that is called acid ash, the chief cause of stomach problems. Foods that are acidic in nature once digested by our bodies are processed foods, refined sugars, whole grains, eggs, dairy products, and meats.

You need to know that a food's alkaline or acid tendency doesn't have anything to do with the pH of the food itself. Limes are acidic in nature but do have an alkalizing effect on our bodies. Alkaline foods are needed to bring our bodies in balance. Like many doctors and experts have said for years, we have to have a meal that is balanced instead of restricting ourselves eating one category of food. Alkaline foods can help counter the risks of acid reflux and acidity, and this will bring us some relief.

**Alkaline Foods You Should Eat**

Alkalizing foods aren't what you think. It turns out that there are some pretty good options out there. Here is a list of the best alkalizing foods that are versatile and delicious. Any of these can be used alongside any other alkalizing vegetable or fruit to help cleanse the body from toxins that are slowly killing us.

· Kale

There is a very good reason why kale has been called the new beef. It is high in vitamin K, calcium, and plant iron. These can help protect you against some cancers. Kale is one of the most alkaline foods out there. Kale is mild in flavor and can kick up any recipe. You can add kale to any smoothie that calls for greens. Add it to soups, salads, and stir-fries for a wonderful alkaline boost.

· Cherries

Cherries are a great source of antioxidants like anthocyanins that can prevent cancer. Studies have shown that cherries can help with inflammation associated with arthritis and joint pain. They could even help prevent cardiovascular disease. Cherries can be put into any smoothie. They are great in a post-workout shake because they contain protein and alkalizing nutrients.

Any post-workout smoothie needs to include alkaline foods because lactic acid gets released when you exercise. Lactic acid helps increase energy. Lactic acid makes the body more acidic; this is why it is important to get rid of acidity by eating more alkaline foods after you exercise.

· Pears

These wonderful fruits are low in sugar but high in fiber. This makes them a wonderful fruit for anyone who has blood sugar problems. They are high in vitamin C, which in turn helps protect cells from carcinogens.

· Zucchini

This is a great source of phytonutrients like lutein. Lutein is in the same antioxidant family as beta carotene, which means it has better benefits for protecting your eyesight. Zucchini is now a very popular vegan, gluten-free, low-carb pasta alternative. Zucchini noodles are easy to make with a spiralizer you can find pretty much anywhere. It is easy to throw together a quick zucchini pasta but pairing it with basil, other spices, and vegetables.

· Strawberries

This is another fruit that is a great source of vitamin C. They also have manganese. Manganese is a trace mineral that helps the body's metabolic function. You can enjoy strawberries in a variety of ways. They can add the smallest amount of sweet to any dish. They are for use in smoothies. Just freeze them, and you won't have to use ice.

· Apples

Apples have always been considered to be the healthiest food around. This is because they are full of antioxidants like vitamin C, detoxifying fiber, and flavonoids that can protect you against cancer.

These nutrients are great for helping with cholesterol and high blood pressure. To get more benefits from your apples, try adding them to dishes you normally wouldn't consider putting them in.

· Watermelon

Watermelons give our bodies essential electrolytes for heart health, like potassium. Because watermelons are made up of mostly water, they can help keep you hydrated better than other vegetables and fruits. Watermelon is a great snack by itself, but it is fun to be creative. Make a smoothie out of watermelon, ginger, agave syrup, and a dash of cayenne.

· Other leafy greens (dandelion, amaranth, turnip, sea vegetables)

Almost all leafy greens have an alkalizing effect on our bodies. It isn't any wonder that our ancestors and doctors always tell us to eat out greens. They have essential minerals needed for our bodies to carry out their functions. You can add sea vegetables, turnip greens, amaranth greens, and dandelion greens to any smoothie or meal.

· Key limes

Most people think that since limes are highly acidic, they have an acidic effect on our bodies, but they are a great alkaline food. Limes are also loaded with vitamin C and can help detoxify our bodies while giving relief from heartburn and acidity.

· Sea salt and seaweed

Sea salt and seaweed have about 12 times more minerals than greens grown in the ground. They are a very alkaline food that can give your body many benefits. You can add in some kelp or nori to your stir fry or soup. Using sea salt as your main seasoning can bring more alkalinity to your body.

· Walnuts

Many people love to munch on walnuts when they feel hunger kick in. Other than being a great source of healthy fats, they create an alkalizing effect in our bodies. Because they are high in calories, you need to limit the amount you eat.

· Onion

Onions, including red onions, are the most important ingredient in Indian cooking, and they bring lots of flavor to your dishes. If you cook them in a healthy oil, like avocado oil, it will increase their alkalinity. Eating them raw is a great choice since onions have many nutritional benefits other than being alkaline-forming. They have antibacterial and anti-inflammatory effects and are full of vitamin C. You can use them in many different ways to spice up your tea, soup, or stir fry.

· Tomatoes

These will be at their most alkalizing when eaten raw. They contain many nutrients, whether raw or cooked. They are full of vitamin C, vitamin B6, and digestive enzymes. Vitamin B6 is very difficult to find naturally. Eat a sliced tomato as a snack with a sprinkle of sea salt, or add it to your favorite omelet or salad.

· Avocado

This is a powerhouse of deliciousness and essential nutrients. Avocados contain lots of healthy fats, plus they are heart-healthy, anti-inflammatory, and very alkalizing.

· Basil

Basil is the tastiest alkalizing ingredient. It is high in calcium, vitamin K, and vitamin A. It is high in flavonoids that have antioxidant effects.

· Mushrooms

Mushrooms contain antioxidants, minerals, vitamins, and protein. They can have many benefits to our health. Antioxidants are chemicals that can help keep our bodies get rid of free radicals. Free radicals are byproducts of bodily processes and metabolism. They get trapped in our bodies, and if too many are trapped, oxidative stress could happen. This could harm the body's cells and could lead to many health problems.

Mushrooms contain choline, vitamin C, and selenium. The antioxidants in mushrooms could help prevent breast, prostate, lung, among other kinds of cancers. Mushrooms can also help with heart health, diabetes, and pregnancy. Mushrooms are high in B vitamins like niacin, pantothenic acid, thiamine, folate, and riboflavin. These help the body form red blood cells and get energy from food.

# Chapter 3:
## *What You Need to Get Started*

### Getting Started as a Beginner

During a detox cleanse, the body and, most importantly, the digestive tract shuts down, allowing the body to focus more on healing because it is no longer using energy to aid digestion. The amount of time you cleanse helps a lot in the healing process, so the longer the fast, the better the results – but it is not the only factor for good results. It's very important to cleanse at least once per year for seven days if you are consuming an alkaline diet. However, Dr. Sebi recommends detoxing for 12 days on smoothies, juice, or raw food.

### How to Make a Good, Natural Smoothie

A common misconception is that fruit and vegetable smoothies are only for healthy and fit people. This couldn't be further from the truth! Everyone - including you - can benefit from drinking a juice or blended drink every day. These drinks can make you feel lighter, cleaner, and with more energy. But not all juices and blends are made equal: some brands contain up to 80% sugar!

Now you might be thinking, "that's too much sugar!" And yeah, it's true that this amount of sugar might not be a great way to start your day if you're trying to lose weight or eat better (especially if the rest of your diet is high in refined carbs!). You see, store-bought juices and smoothies are often loaded with sugar, even if they say "100%

natural" or "organic". And this is a shame because it means that people with a sweet tooth are choosing over-sweetened juices and smoothies instead of eating fresh fruit.

Without getting too technical, let me explain why store-bought juice and smoothies tend to be sugary. Many brands of juice include added sugar in the form of high fructose corn syrup (HFCS), a highly refined starch made from genetically modified corn. HFCS is cheap and easy to use, but it also contains very few vitamins and minerals compared to real fruit.

Now some people prefer the taste of hydrogenated oils (trans fats) that are formed when liquid vegetable oil is put through high-pressure processing techniques. Trans fats are actually better tasting than hydrogenated oils because they stay liquid at room temperature - you won't notice when you drink a smoothie that has one tablespoon of trans fat in it. Foods that contain trans-fat include doughnuts, French fries, waffles, cakes, cookies, and frosting.

Several brands of juices and smoothies use "natural" sweeteners like honey, agave syrup, or maple syrup. These sweeteners are known to be high in fructose and cause the body to absorb them more quickly. Is it a coincidence that recent studies have found that children with high levels of fructose in their blood there are more likely to have obesity, type 2 diabetes, and metabolic theory?

If you want to enjoy healthy fruit smoothies without all the sugar, you need a way to get real fruit into your diet and detoxify your system at the same time. So how do you know which fruit is actually good for your health? First of all, you'll need to find a source that has all the vitamins and minerals you need to keep your body running smoothly. Remember that nature-designed fruits with all their various nutrients to work together; combining fruits in a smoothie helps you get a great balance of vitamins and minerals. This is especially important if you're eating lots of fresh produce while on a juice cleanse diet.

**How to Get the Right Herbs**

A lot of people ask what are the best herbs. There are things to consider when choosing herbs for your kitchen. I've put together some information on how to get the right ones and different ways you can use them in your cooking.

Some people like using fresh herbs, while others prefer dry herbs because they last longer. I think it all depends on the kind of herbs you use in cooking. Most people prefer to have fresh herbs, but they are actually harder to find than dried herbs. If you want fresh herbs, you need to grow them yourself or buy them at a local grocery or farmer's market if they are seasonal. The best time to get them is around the end of summer when they are still in season and at their freshest.

Dried herbs are easier to find and store. You can buy dried herbs in the spice section of most supermarkets or in health food stores. They usually come in small bottles. Get your hands on the containers that come with shaker tops so you can shake them into your cooking pots. When buying dried herbs, it is important to check if they are organic. If you don't, you'll be adding all kinds of pesticides and chemicals into your cooking as well. No one wants to do that.

**What to Expect During the Smoothie Detox?**

- cold and flu symptoms

- changes in bowel movements
- fatigue and low energy
- difficulty sleeping
- itching
- headaches
- muscle aches and pains
- acne. rashes and breakouts
- mucus expels (catarrh, etc.)
- lower blood pressure

These symptoms are only temporary and usually resolve after the first one to two weeks.

## How to Break Your Smoothie Detox Fast

Slowly reintroduce solids: if you are doing water or a liquid fast, you will need to slowly reintroduce solid foods. Begin by introducing solids like high water-content fruits. These include watermelon, apples, and berries. Thereafter, you can proceed to introduce softer fruit solids like bananas and avocados. Later, you can incorporate harder solids like veggies. All foods must be listed on the nutrition guide. However, if doing a fruit or raw veggie fast, you can break the fast right away on solid foods. Drink one gallon spring water daily together with revitalizing herbs and sea moss.

# Tips to Motivate You to Get Started

## Smoothie Cleanse: Tips And Advice

If you want to do a cleanse, be ready for the food and energy fluctuation. A cleanse diet will change your lifestyle, especially you're eating habits. You might feel hunger, headaches, and changes in energy levels while you get used to the detox changes.

Don't be afraid to experiment. You don't have to drink only one green smoothie during the diet. Find new recipes and mix different fruit and vegetables to get the best for you. As a result, you won't get bored and will enjoy your smoothies.

Make a smoothie schedule. It's a good habit to have systematic eating, specifically while you on a smoothie cleanse diet. Start with your favorite vegetable smoothie in the morning.

Weight loss and cleansing aren't the same things. The real purpose of a detox diet is to reduce the number of toxins in your body, and weight loss is a side effect. This diet even changes our taste buds. It means you will want less junk food and more healthy food.

Listening to your body while doing a detox cleanse. You shouldn't feel bad and suffer during the diet. Watch how your body reacts, have a good rest, and if you are extra hungry get some healthy snacks like fresh vegetables with hummus or something similar. If you have a headache, drink more water. Try to comfort your body! It might be that you feel really horrible on the first or second day of detoxing. It means you have to stop your detox for a little break and wait for the right time to cleanse your body.

Stay hydrated! It's important not only for any diet but and for a healthy lifestyle too. While you cleanse your body, you need to release the toxins from the body, and the water is the best helper! It will improve the elimination process and prevent dehydration, which is especially dangerous while you are on a detox or cleanse diet. Try to drink about 2-3 liters each day during the cleanse.

Sleep well during the diet. Your body is working hard, so you need to have extra rest. It's better to sleep at least 8 hours at night and take a short nap during the day if you feel tired.

Don't be upset if something doesn't go as planned. It's not a reason to stop or give up, so get back in the game and go on your cleanse. It's alright if you have missed a meal or take a day off, especially if you need it. Just keep moving!

Avoid any stress and let your mind have a rest too. Try not to overload your schedule with commitments or appointments; give yourself time to relax and do what you like.

# Chapter 4:
# **Smoothies Recipes**

### 1. **Avocado Blueberry Smoothie**

Preparation Time: 5 minutes

Cooking Time: 5 minutes

Servings: 1

Ingredients:

- 1 tsp. chia seeds
- ½ cup unsweetened coconut milk
- 1 avocado
- ½ cup blueberries

Directions:

1. Add all Ingredients to the blender and blend until smooth and creamy.
2. Serve immediately and enjoy.

Nutrition:

Calories: 389

Fat: 34.6g.

Carbs: 20.7g.

Protein: 4.8g.

Fiber: 0g.

## 2. Veggie-Ful Smoothie

Preparation Time: 5 minutes
Cooking Time: 0 minutes
Servings: 2
Ingredients:
- 1 cup spring water, chilled
- ½ of a large avocado
- 2 large pears; cored, seeded
- 1 cup watercress, fresh
- 1 large cucumber; peeled, seeded
- 1 cup Romaine lettuce, fresh
- 2 Medjool dates, pitted

Directions:

1) Use a high-power blender and place all the ingredients in the order of the list.

2) Cover the jar of the blender and then pulse at high speed for 30–60 seconds or more until the smoothie liquid is fully circulating.

3) Let the smoothie cool in the refrigerator until ready to drink or serve straight away over ice cubes.

Nutrition:
Calories: 283
Carbs: 56 g
Fat: 5.3 g
Protein: 2.8 g

## 3. Detox Sugar Smoothie

Preparation Time: 5 minutes
Cooking Time: 0 minutes
Servings: 2
Ingredients:

- 2 cups soft-jelly coconut milk; unsweetened, homemade
- 1 large avocado, pitted
- 2 key limes, juiced
- 1 ½ cup dandelion greens, fresh
- 2 teaspoons bromide plus powder

Directions:

1) Plug in a high-power blender and then place all the ingredients in the order of the list.
2) Cover the blender and pulse at high speed for 30–60 seconds or more until the smoothie liquid is fully circulating within the jar.
3) Let the smoothie cool in the refrigerator until ready to drink or serve straight away over ice cubes.

Nutrition:
Calories: 195
Carbs: 14.1 g
Fat: 14.3 g
Protein: 2.4 g

## 4. Walnut Milk and Dandelion Smoothie

Preparation Time: 5 minutes
Cooking Time: 0 minutes
Servings: 2
Ingredients:

- 2 ½ cups walnut milk; unsweetened, homemade
- ½ of a large avocado, pitted
- 4 cups dandelion greens, fresh
- 2/3 cup zucchini, diced
- 6 tablespoons hemp seeds

Directions:
1) Plug in a high-power blender and then place all the ingredients in the order of the list.
2) Cover the jar of the blender with its lid and then pulse at high speed for 30–60 seconds or more until the smoothie liquid is fully circulating.
3) Let the smoothie cool in the refrigerator until ready to drink or serve straight away over ice cubes.

Nutrition:
Calories: 443
Carbs: 22.2 g
Fat: 33 g
Protein: 14.4 g

## 5. Blueberry Pie Smoothie

Preparation Time: 5 minutes
Cooking Time: 0 minutes
Servings: 2
Ingredients:

- 4 cups soft-jelly coconut milk; unsweetened, homemade
- 2 tablespoons walnut butter, homemade
- ½ cup amaranth, cooked
- 2 cups blueberries, fresh
- 4 medium burro bananas, peeled
- 2 teaspoons bromide plus powder
- 4 tablespoons date sugar

Directions:
1) Plug in a high-power blender and then place all the ingredients in the order of the list.
2) Cover the jar of the blender with its lid and then pulse at high speed for 30–60 seconds or more until the smoothie liquid is fully circulating within the jar.
3) Let the smoothie cool in the refrigerator until ready to drink or serve straight away over ice cubes.

Nutrition:
Calories: 534
Carbs: 81.4 g
Fat: 20.2 g
Protein: 6.7 g

## 6. Lettuce, Blueberry, and Coconut Smoothie

Preparation Time: 5 minutes
Cooking Time: 0 minutes
Servings: 2
Ingredients:

- 1 cup coconut water; unsweetened, chilled
- 1 cup ginger tea, brewed
- 2 cups Romaine lettuce, fresh
- 1 medium burro banana, peeled
- ½ cup blueberries, fresh
- 4 tablespoons key lime juice

Directions:

1) Plug in a high-power blender and then place all the ingredients in the order of the list.

2) Cover the jar of the blender with its lid and then pulse at high speed for 30–60 seconds or more until the smoothie liquid is fully circulating.

3) Let the smoothie cool in the refrigerator until ready to drink or serve straight away over ice cubes.

Nutrition:
Calories: 161
Carbs: 36.6 g
Fat: 0.7 g
Protein: 2 g

## 7. Kale Banana Smoothie

Preparation Time: 5 minutes
Cooking Time: 5 minutes
Servings: 2
Ingredients:
- 2 cups of kale (chopped)
- 2/3 cup of bananas (sliced)
- 1/4 cup of milk
- 1/3 cup of orange juice
- 1 tablespoon of flax seed meal
- 1 tablespoon of coconut oil

Directions:
1. Add 2 cups of chopped kale, 2/3 cup of sliced bananas, 1/4 cup of milk, 1/3 cup of orange juice, 1 tablespoon of flax seed meal, and 1 tablespoon of coconut oil in a blender or food processor and combine. If you want it a little more frozen, add a couple of ice cubes to the blender.

Nutrition:
Calories- 239
Fat-1 g
Protein- 3 g
Carbs-15 g

## 8. Vanilla Spinach, Banana, Grape and Apple Smoothie

Preparation Time: 5 minutes
Cooking Time: 5 minutes
Servings: 2
Ingredients:

- 1 1/2 cups of spinach (fresh)
- 1 cup of grapes (seedless, purple or green)
- 3/4 cup of yogurt (vanilla)
- 2/3 cup of banana (sliced)
- 1/3 cup of apples (cored, peeled, chopped)

Directions:

1. Add 1 1/2 cups of fresh spinach, 1 cup of seedless grapes, 3/4 cup of vanilla yogurt, 2/3 cup of sliced banana, and 1/3 cup of chopped apples to a blender or food processor. Combine until smooth.

Nutrition:
Calories- 239
Fat-1 g
Protein- 3 g
Carbs-15 g

## 9. Ginger Avocado, Apple, Carrot, Kale Smoothie

Preparation Time: 5 minutes
Cooking Time: 5 minutes
Servings: 2
Ingredients:
- 1 avocado (peeled, pitted)
- 1 lemon (peeled)
- 1 kale leaf
- 2 cups of water (cold)
- 2/3 cup of apples (cored, peeled, chopped)
- 1/2 cup of parsley (fresh)
- 1/2 cup of carrots (chunked)
- 1 tablespoon of flax seeds
- 1 1/4 teaspoon of ginger (ground)
- 2 ice cubes

Directions:
1. Add peeled and pitted avocado, 1 peeled lemon, 1 kale leaf, 2 cups of cold water, 2/3 cup of cored, peeled, and chopped apples, 1/2 cup of fresh parsley, 1/2 cup of chunked carrots, 1 tablespoon of flax seeds, 1 1/4 teaspoon of ground ginger, and 2 ice cubes to a blender or food processor and combine until smooth.

Nutrition:
Calories- 239
Fat-1 g
Protein- 3 g
Carbs-15 g

## 10. Spinach Peanut Butter Smoothie

Preparation Time: 5 minutes

Cooking Time: 5 minutes

Servings: 2

Ingredients:
- 2 cups of spinach
- 1 cup of milk
- 1 cup of ice cubes
- 1/2 cup of yogurt (plain)
- 2/3 cup of bananas (sliced, frozen)
- 1 tablespoon of peanut butter (creamy)

Directions:
1. Add the 2 cups of spinach, 1 cup of milk, 1 cup of ice cubes, 1/2 cup of plain yogurt, 2/3 cup of frozen sliced bananas, and 1 tablespoon of creamy peanut butter to a blender or food processor and combine until nice and smooth.

Nutrition:

Calories- 239

Fat-1 g

Protein- 3 g

Carbs-15 g

## 11. Rhubarb, Banana, Cranberry Smoothie

Preparation Time: 5 minutes

Cooking Time: 5 minutes

Servings: 2

Ingredients:

- 1 cup of rhubarb (frozen, chopped)
- 1 cup of cranberry juice (used blended juice if desired)
- 2/3 cup of bananas (frozen, sliced)
- 1/2 cup of yogurt (vanilla)

Directions:

1. Add the 1 cup of frozen, chopped rhubarb, 1 cup of cranberry juice, 2/3 cup of frozen, sliced bananas, and 1/2 cup of vanilla yogurt to a blender or food processor and combine until smooth.

Nutrition:

Calories- 239

Fat-1 g

Protein- 3 g

Carbs-15 g

## 12. Cinnamon Apple, Pear, Spinach Smoothie

Preparation Time: 5 minutes

Cooking Time: 5 minutes

Servings: 2

Ingredients:

- 1 pear (peeled, cored, sliced)
- 1 cup of apple juice
- 1 cup of spinach (fresh)
- 1/2 cup of ice
- 1/2 cup of yogurt (plain)
- 1 teaspoon of cinnamon (ground)

Directions:

1. Add 1 peeled, cored, and sliced pear, 1 cup of apple juice, 1 cup of fresh spinach, 1/2 cup of ice, 1/2 cup of plain yogurt, and 1 teaspoon of ground cinnamon to a blender or food processor and combine until smooth.

Nutrition:

Calories- 239

Fat-1 g

Protein- 3 g

Carbs-15 g

## 13. Honeydew, Grapes, Cucumber, Broccoli Smoothie

Preparation Time: 5 minutes

Cooking Time: 5 minutes

Servings: 2

Ingredients:

- 3/4 cup of honeydew melon (peeled, seeded, chopped)
- 3/4 cup of ice cubes
- 1/4 cup of green grapes (seedless)
- 1/4 cup of cucumber (peeled, chopped)
- 2 tablespoons of broccoli florets
- 1/4 of a sprig of mint (fresh leaves)

Directions:

1. Add 3/4 cup of peeled, seeded, and chopped honeydew melon, 3/4 cup of ice cubes, 1/4 cup of seedless green grapes, 1/4 cup of peeled and chopped cucumber, 2 tablespoons of broccoli florets, and 1/4 fresh sprig of mint to a blender or food processor and combine until smooth.

Nutrition:

Calories- 239

Fat-1 g

Protein- 3 g

Carbs-15 g

## 14. Minty Melon Smoothie

Preparation Time: 5 minutes
Cooking Time: 5 minutes
Servings: 2
Ingredients:

- 1/2 English cucumber (hothouse cucumber - chopped)
- 4 sprigs of mint (fresh leaves)
- 1 cup of honeydew melon (chopped)
- 1 cup of passion fruit juice
- 1 cup of ice

Directions:

1. Add 1/2 of a chopped English cucumber, 4 sprigs of fresh mint leaves only, 1 cup of chopped honeydew melon, 1 cup of passion fruit juice, and 1 cup of ice to blender or food processor and combine until smooth.

Nutrition:
Calories- 239
Fat-1 g
Protein- 3 g
Carbs-15 g

## 15. Orange Banana Green Smoothie

Preparation Time: 5 minutes

Cooking Time: 5 minutes

Servings: 2

Ingredients:

- 2 bananas (peeled, ripe)
- 1 orange (peeled, quartered)
- 1 kale leaf (torn)
- 1 cup of ice water (water and ice)

Directions:

1. Add 2 peeled ripe bananas, 1 peeled and quartered orange, 1 ripped into pieces kale leaf, with 1 cup of ice water into a blender or food processor and combine until smooth.

Nutrition:

Calories- 239

Fat-1 g

Protein- 3 g

Carbs-15 g

## 16. Orange Zucchini Smoothie

Preparation Time: 5 minutes
Cooking Time: 5 minutes
Servings: 2
Ingredients:
- 1 zucchini (cubed)
- 1 cup of orange juice
- 1/4 cup of ice cubes
- 2 tablespoons of honey
- 3/4 teaspoons of vanilla extract

Directions:
1. Add 1 cubed zucchini, 1 cup of orange juice, 1/4 cup of ice cubes, 2 tablespoons of honey, and 3/4 teaspoons of vanilla extract into a blender or food processor and combine until smooth.

Nutrition:
Calories- 239
Fat-1 g
Protein- 3 g
Carbs-15 g

## 17. Fruity Herbal Tea Smoothie

Preparation Time: 5 minutes

Cooking Time: 0 minutes

Servings: 2

Ingredients:
- 2 cups Dr. Sebi's herbal tea; brewed, cooled
- 2 key limes, juiced
- 2 tablespoons coconut oil
- 2 tablespoons agave syrup
- 2 Seville oranges, peeled
- 1 large mango; peeled, destoned

Directions:

1) Plug in a high-power blender and then place all the ingredients in the order of the list.

2) Cover the jar of the blender and then pulse at high speed for 30–60 seconds or more until the smoothie liquid is fully circulating.

3) Let the smoothie cool in the refrigerator until ready to drink or serve straight away over ice cubes.

Nutrition:

Calories: 396.5

Carbs: 63.5 g

Fat: 14.5 g

Protein: 3 g

## 18. Cucumber Smoothie

Preparation Time: 2 minutes

Cooking Time: 0 minutes

Servings: 1

Ingredients:

- ½ piece of cucumber
- 2 pieces of limes
- 80 ml of water
- 20 g lamb's lettuce
- 1 tbsp walnuts

Directions:

1. Peel and roughly chop the cucumber and remove the peel from the limes.
2. Put all ingredients in the blender and mix for approx. 2 minutes
3. Pour the healthy smoothie into a glass and enjoy.

Nutrition:

Calories: 208 kcal

Carbohydrates: 7 g

of which sugar: 2 g

Fat: 13 g

Protein: 5 g

## 19. Swiss Chard Smoothie

Preparation Time: 2 minutes
Cooking Time: 0 minutes
Servings: 1
Ingredients:
- 80 g Swiss chard
- 40 g Greek yogurt
- 80 ml orange juice
- 1 tbsp pumpkin seeds
- 1 teaspoon honey

Directions:
1. Wash the chard and spin dry.
2. Put washed chard with the remaining ingredients in a blender and mix well.
3. Pour the creamy smoothie into a glass or take away bottle and drink.

Nutrition:
Calories: 199 kcal
Carbohydrates: 32 g
of which sugar: 17 g
Fat: 4 g
Protein: 9 g

## 20. Mint Smoothie

Preparation Time: 2 minutes
Cooking Time: 0 minutes
Servings: 1
Ingredients:
- ½ bunch of mint
- 100 ml of water
- 2 tbsp roasted walnuts
- 1 tbsp maple syrup
- 1 squirt of lemon juice
- 1 pinch of grated ginger

Directions:
1. Pluck the mint leaves from the stems, wash and spin dry.
2. Put all ingredients in the blender, pour into a glass and enjoy.

Nutrition:
Calories: 387 kcal
Carbohydrates: 33 g
of which sugar: 0 g
Fat: 25 g
Protein: 0 g

## 21. Zucchini and Dill Smoothie

Preparation Time: 2 minutes
Cooking Time: 0 minutes
Servings: 1
Ingredients:
- 1 zucchini
- 100 ml hazelnut milk
- 1 tbsp dill
- 1 tbsp hazelnut puree
- 1 pinch of nutmeg

Directions:
1. Peel the zucchini and cut into large pieces.
2. Put all ingredients in a blender and mix into a creamy shake.
3. Pour the creamy smoothie into a glass and drink.

Nutrition:
Calories: 233 kcal
Carbohydrates: 14 g
of which sugar: 9 g
Fat: 17 g
Protein: 6 g

## 22. Kiwi and Lemon Smoothie

Preparation Time: 5 minutes
Cooking Time: 0 minutes
Servings: 1
Ingredients:
- 2 pcs. kiwi fruit
- 1 piece of lemon
- 3 tbsp yogurt
- 1 tbsp elderflower syrup

Directions:
1. Remove the peel from the lemon and kiwi fruit and cut into large pieces.
2. Put all the ingredients in a blender and process into a healthy shake.
3. Pour smoothie into a glass and enjoy.

Nutrition:
Calories: 230 kcal
Carbohydrates: 44 g
of which sugar: 23 g
Fat: 2 g
Protein: 8 g

## 23. Apple, Walnut, and Green Smoothie

Preparation Time: 5 minutes

Cooking Time: 0 minutes

Servings: 2

Ingredients:

- 2 cups walnut milk; unsweetened, homemade
- 1 tablespoon agave syrup
- 1 cup turnip greens, fresh
- 1 cup watercress, fresh
- 2 medium apples; fresh, cored, seeded
- 2 cups blueberries, unsweetened
- ½ cup Brazil nuts, unsalted

Directions:

1) Plug in a high-power blender and place all the ingredients in the order of the list.

2) Cover the blender and then pulse at high speed for 30–60 seconds or more until the smoothie liquid is fully circulating.

3) Let the smoothie cool in the refrigerator until ready to drink or serve straight away over ice cubes.

Nutrition:

Calories: 571.5

Carbs: 61.4 g

Fat: 32.4 g

Protein: 8.6 g

## 24. Pineapple Coconut Detox Smoothie

Preparation Time: 5 minutes

Cooking Time: 5 minutes

Servings: 2

Ingredients:

- 4 cups of kale, chopped
- 2 cups of coconut water
- 2 bananas
- 2 cups of pineapple

Directions:

1. Add all listed ingredients into a blender.
2. Blend until a smooth and creamy texture.
3. Serve chilled and enjoy!

Nutrition:

Calories: 299

Fat: 1.1 g

Carbohydrates: 71.5g

Protein: 7.9g

## 25. Avocado Detox Smoothie

Preparation Time: 5 minutes

Cooking Time: 5 minutes

Servings: 2

Ingredients:

- 4 cups of spinach, chopped
- 1 avocado, chopped
- 3 cups of apple juice
- 2apples, unpeeled, cored and chopped

Directions:

1. Add all the listed Ingredients into a blender.
2. Blend until you have a smooth and creamy texture.
3. Serve chilled and enjoy!

Nutrition:

Calories: 336

Fat: 13.8g

Carbohydrates: 55.8g

Protein: 3g

## 26. Chamomile Ginger Detox Smoothie

Preparation Time: 5 minutes

Cooking Time: 5 minutes

Servings: 2

Ingredients:

- 3 tablespoons of collard greens
- 1 tablespoon of chamomile flowers, dried
- 1 pear, chopped
- 1 cantaloupe, sliced and chopped
- ½ inch ginger root, peeled
- ½ lemon, juiced
- 1 cup of ice
- 1 cup of water

Directions:

1. Add all the listed ingredients into a blender.
2. Blend until smooth.
3. Serve chilled and enjoy!

Nutrition:

Calories: 86

Fat: 0g

Carbohydrates: 22g

Protein: 2g

## 27. Wheatgrass Detox Smoothie

Preparation Time: 5 minutes
Cooking Time: 5 minutes
Servings: 2
Ingredients:

- 3 tablespoons of Swiss chard
- 1 banana, peeled
- 3 tablespoons of almonds
- 1 teaspoon of wheatgrass powder
- 2 kiwis, peeled
- 1 cup of ice
- 1 cup of water

Directions:

1. Add all the ingredients into a blender, except kiwis
2. Blend until smooth
3. Add kiwis and blend again
4. Serve chilled and enjoy!

Nutrition:
Calories: 154
Fat: 6g
Carbohydrates: 24g
Protein: 4g

## 28. Charcoal Lemonade Detox Smoothie

Preparation Time: 5 minutes

Cooking Time: 5 minutes

Servings: 2

Ingredients:

- 3 tablespoons of collard green
- ½ teaspoon of charcoal activated
- 1 apple, chopped
- 1 lemon, peeled
- ½ inch ginger root
- 1 cucumber, chopped
- 1 cup of ice
- 1 cup of water

Directions:

1. Add all the ingredients into a blender.
2. Blend until smooth.
3. Serve chilled and enjoy!

Nutrition:

Calories: 88

Fat: 0.6g

Carbohydrates: 23g

Protein: 2g

## 29. Banana Oatmeal Detox Smoothie

Preparation Time: 5 minutes

Cooking Time: 5 minutes

Servings: 2

Ingredients:

- 3 tablespoons of collard greens
- 3 tablespoons of oats
- 1 banana, peeled
- 1 apple, chopped
- 1 teaspoon of cinnamon
- 1 cup of ice
- 1 cup of water

Directions:

1. Add all the listed ingredients into a blender.
2. Blend until you have a smooth and creamy texture.
3. Serve chilled and enjoy!

Nutrition:

Calories: 162

Fat: 1 g

Carbohydrates: 41 g

Protein: 3g

## 30. Apple Chia Detox Smoothie

Preparation Time: 5 minutes

Cooking Time: 5 minutes

Servings: 2

Ingredients:

- 3 tablespoons of collard greens
- 1 mini cucumber
- 1 tablespoon of chia seeds
- 4 kumquats
- 1 apple, chopped
- ½ teaspoon of chia seeds
- 1 cup of ice
- 1 cup of water

Directions:

1. Add all the listed ingredients to a blender.
2. Blend until you have a smooth and creamy texture.
3. Serve chilled and enjoy!

Nutrition:

Calories: 108

Fat: 2g

Carbohydrates: 21 g

Protein: 3g

## 31. Dandelion Greens and Mixed Berry Smoothie

Preparation Time: 5 minutes

Cooking Time: 5 minutes

Servings: 2

Ingredients:
- honey (.5 t)
- frozen blackberries (1 c)
- coconut oil (1 t)
- flax seed (1 t)
- frozen banana (1 peeled)
- cinnamon (.25 tsp)
- coconut oil (1 t)
- water (1 c)
- dandelion greens (1 c)

Directions:

1. This recipe can be ready in 5 minutes, makes 1 serving (24 oz.), and will take approximately 45 seconds of blending, assuming you are using a blender of 1000 watts.

Nutrition:

270 Calories

15 g of fat

9 g of fat (saturated)

36 g of carbs

75 mg of sodium

7 g of fiber

19 g of sugar

18 g of protein

## 32. Baby Spinach and Pear Smoothie

Preparation Time: 5 minutes

Cooking Time: 5 minutes

Servings: 2

Ingredients:

- pear (1 peeled)
- flax seed (1 t)
- baby spinach (1 c)
- water (1 c)
- ginger (.5 tsp)
- honey (.5 t)
- water (1 c)
- flax seed (1 t)

Directions:

1. This recipe can be ready in 5 minutes, makes 1 serving (24 oz.), and will take approximately 45 seconds of blending. assuming you are using a blender of 1000 watts.

Nutrition:

222 Calories

8 g of fat

0 g of fat (saturated)

39 g of carbs

24 mg of sodium

8 g of fiber

26 g of sugar

3 g of protein

## 33. Spicy Spinach Smoothie

Preparation Time: 5 minutes
Cooking Time: 5 minutes
Servings: 2
Ingredients:
- frozen banana (1 peeled)
- coconut oil (.5 t)
- honey (.5 t)
- chili powder (.25 tsp)
- water (1 c)
- spinach (1 c)
- cayenne pepper (.25 tsp)
- flax seed (1 t)

Directions:

1. This recipe can be ready in 5 minutes, makes 1 serving (24 oz.), and will take approximately 45 seconds of blending, assuming you are using a blender of 1000 watts.

Nutrition:
170 Calories
8 g of fat
1 g of fat (saturated)
28 g of carbs
300 mg of sodium
4 g of fiber
15 g of sugar
2 g of protein

## 34. Romaine Lettuce and Ginger Smoothie

Preparation Time: 5 minutes

Cooking Time: 5 minutes

Servings: 2

Ingredients:
- Romaine lettuce (3 c)
- ginger (.25 inches)
- frozen mango (1 pitted)
- lemons (2 peeled)
- chia seeds (2 t)
- spinach (2 c)
- water (1 c)

Directions:

1. This recipe can be ready in 5 minutes, makes 1 serving (32 oz.), and will take approximately 45 seconds of blending, assuming you are using a blender of 1000 watts.

Nutrition:

135 Calories

4 g of fat

0 g of fat (saturated)

60 g of carbs

85 mg of sodium

1 g of fiber

24 g of sugar

9 g of protein

## 35. Peach Yogurt Smoothie

Preparation Time: 5 minutes

Cooking Time: 5 minutes

Servings: 2

Ingredients:

- 1/2 banana
- 1 1/2 cups cubed peaches
- 1 cup vanilla yogurt
- ¼ cup orange juice
- 1 teaspoon honey

Directions:

1. Place all the ingredients in a blender and blend until smooth.
2. Pour into two glasses and serve as a quick breakfast for you and a friend, or refrigerate one serving and take the other in a travel mug on the go.

Nutrition:

Calories- 239

Fat-1 g

Protein- 3 g

Carbs-15 g

## 36. Creamy Carrot Smoothie

Preparation Time: 5 minutes
Cooking Time: 5 minutes
Servings: 2
Ingredients:
- 5 large carrots
- 1 tablespoon lemon juice
- ¼ cup orange juice
- 1/2 cup nonfat yogurt
- 1/2 cup skim milk

Directions:
1. In a blender or food processor grate the carrots. Separate the grated carrot from the juice using a fine strainer. Reserve the juice.
2. Place the grated carrot, lemon juice, orange juice, yogurt, and skim milk in a blender and blend until smooth.
3. Blend in the reserved carrot juice. Pour into a tall glass.

Nutrition:
Calories- 320
Fat-1 g
Protein- 3 g
Carbs-19 g

## 37. Blackberry Apple Smoothie

Preparation Time: 5 minutes

Cooking Time: 5 minutes

Servings: 1

Ingredients:

- 1 cup blackberries
- 1 apple, sliced
- 1 cup nonfat yogurt
- 1/2 cup skim milk

Directions:

1. Combine all the ingredients in a blender until smooth. Pour into a tall glass.

Nutrition:

Calories- 298

Fat-1 g

Protein- 2 g,

Carbs-15 g

## 38. Fruit Medley Smoothie

Preparation Time: 5 minutes

Cooking Time: 5 minutes

Servings: 1

Ingredients:

- ¼ cup blueberries
- ¼ cup fresh strawberries
- 1 large peach, sliced
- 1 cup raspberries
- 1/2 cup nonfat yogurt
- 1/2 cup skim milk

Directions:

1. Combine all the ingredients in a blender until smooth. Pour into a tall glass.

Nutrition:

Calories- 268

Fat- 2g

Protein- 3 g

Carbs- 10 g

## 39. Papaya and Quinoa Smoothie

Preparation Time: 5 minutes
Cooking Time: 0 minutes
Servings: 2
Ingredients:

- 2 cups hemp milk; unsweetened, homemade
- 1 cup quinoa, cooked
- 2 cups papaya; fresh, cubed
- 2 Medjool dates, pitted
- 2 teaspoon bromide plus powder

Directions:

1) Plug in a high-power blender and then place all ingredients in the order of the ingredients list.
2) Cover the jar of the blender with its lid and then pulse at high speed for 30–60 seconds or more until the smoothie liquid is fully circulating within the jar.
3) Let the smoothie cool in the refrigerator until ready to drink or serve straight away over ice cubes.

Nutrition:
Calories: 348
Carbs: 61 g
Fat: 8.5 g
Protein: 7.8 g

## 40. Choco Collards

Preparation Time: 5 minutes

Cooking Time: 5 minutes

Servings: 2

Ingredients:

- 1 cup collards
- 3 tsps. cocoa powder
- 1 tsp. cinnamon
- 1 banana

Directions:

1. Clean blender before use.

2. Now add all ingredient: together and blend it for two minutes

3. That's it. Enjoy.

Nutrition:

Calories- 239

Fat-1 g

Protein- 3 g

Carbs-15 g

## 41. Peach Green Smoothie

Preparation Time: 5 minutes

Cooking Time: 5 minutes

Servings: 2

Ingredients:

- peach, pealed
- 1 tsp, cinnamon
- 1 cup spinach
- 1 cup arugula
- 1 cup water

Directions:

1. Blend spinach and arugula together.
2. Add all the other ingredient into the blender and blend again.
3. Use two cubes of ice to make the smoothie cold.
4. That's it. Enjoy.

Nutrition:

Calories- 239

Fat-1 g

Protein- 3 g

Carbs-15 g

## 42. Choy Choco

Preparation Time: 5 minutes
Cooking Time: 5 minutes
Servings: 2
Ingredients:

- 1 cup coconut water
- 1 tsp. cinnamon
- 1/2 cup cherries (with pits removed)
- 1 cup bok choy, sliced
- 1 cup spinach

Directions:

1. Take the spinach and coconut water and blend together.
2. Add the other ingredients in the blender and blend again.
4. Enjoy.

Nutrition:
Calories- 239
Fat-1 g
Protein- 3 g
Carbs-15 g

## 43. Parsley with Mixed Cherry Smoothie

Preparation Time: 5 minutes

Cooking Time: 5 minutes

Servings: 2

Ingredients:

- 1 cup parsley
- 1 cup mixed berry
- 1 cup water
- 2 tsp honey
- 1 cup broccoli

Directions:

1. Always keep blender clean.
2. Now add all ingredients into the blender and blend.
3. That's it. Enjoy.

Nutrition:

Calories- 239

Fat-1 g

Protein- 3 g

Carbs-15 g

## 44. Apple Berry Green Smoothie

Preparation Time: 5 minutes
Cooking Time: 5 minutes
Servings: 2
Ingredients:
- 2 apples (cored, peeled, chopped)
- 2 bananas (frozen, peeled, sliced)
- 2 cups of spinach (fresh baby)
- 1 cup of carrots (peeled, chopped)
- 1 cup of orange juice
- 1 cup of strawberries (frozen)
- 1 cup of ice

Directions:
1. Add 2 cored, peeled, chopped apples, 2 frozen, peeled, sliced bananas, 2 cups of fresh baby spinach, 1 cup of peeled, chopped carrots, 1 cup of orange juice, 1 cup of frozen strawberries, and 1 cup of ice into a blender or food processor and combine until smooth.

Nutrition:
Calories- 239
Fat-1 g
Protein- 3 g
Carbs-15 g

## 45. Strawberry Banana Green Smoothie

Preparation Time: 5 minutes
Cooking Time: 5 minutes
Servings: 2
Ingredients:
- 2 cups of spinach
- 2 cups of strawberries (frozen)
- 2/3 cup of banana (frozen, sliced)
- 1/2 cup of ice
- 2 tablespoons of honey

Directions:
1. Add 2 cups of spinach, 2 cups of frozen strawberries, 2/3 cup of frozen sliced banana, 1/2 cup of ice, and 2 tablespoons of honey into a blender or food processor and combine until smooth.

Nutrition:
Calories- 239
Fat-1 g
Protein- 3 g
Carbs-15 g

## 46. Maple, Banana, Kale Smoothie

Preparation Time: 5 minutes

Cooking Time: 5 minutes

Servings: 2

Ingredients:
- 2 cups of kale (chopped)
- 2/3 cup of banana (sliced)
- 1/2 cup of milk
- 1 tablespoon of flax seeds
- 1 teaspoon of honey

Directions:
1. Add 2 cups of chopped kale, 2/3 cup of sliced banana, 1/2 cup of milk, 1 tablespoon of flax seeds, and 1 teaspoon of honey into a blender or food processor and combine until smooth.

Nutrition:

Calories- 239

Fat-1 g

Protein- 3 g

Carbs-15 g

## 47. Tropical Kiwi Green Smoothie

Preparation Time: 5 minutes

Cooking Time: 5 minutes

Servings: 2

Ingredients:

- 1/2 kiwi (peeled, sliced)
- 1/4 cup of pineapple (chunked)
- 1/4 cup of grapes (seedless, green)
- 1/4 cup of mango (peeled, seeded, chunked)
- 1/4 cup of spinach
- 1/4 cup of ice water (water and ice)

Directions:

1. Add 1/2 peeled, sliced kiwi, 1/4 cup of chunked pineapple, 1/4 cup of seedless green grapes, 1/4 cup of peeled, seeded, chunked mango, 1/4 cup of spinach, 1/4 cup of ice water into a blender or food processor and combine until smooth.

Nutrition:

Calories- 239

Fat-1 g

Protein- 3 g

Carbs-15 g

## 48. Tropical Green Kiwi Smoothie II

Preparation Time: 5 minutes
Cooking Time: 5 minutes
Servings: 2
Ingredients:
- 1/2 kiwi (peeled)
- 1/2 cup of apple (peeled, cored, chopped)
- 1/2 cup of pineapples (chopped)
- 1/2 cup of ice cubes
- 1/2 cup of carrots (chopped)
- 1/3 cup of bananas (sliced)

Directions:
1. Add 1/2 peeled kiwi, 1/2 cup of peeled, cored, chopped apple, 1/2 cup of chopped pineapples, 1/2 cup of ice cubes, 1/2 cup of chopped carrots and 1/3 cup of sliced bananas into a blender or food processor and combine until smooth.

Nutrition:
Calories- 239
Fat-1 g
Protein- 3 g
Carbs-15 g

## 49. Celery with Orange Smoothie

Preparation Time: 5 minutes
Cooking Time: 5 minutes
Servings: 2
Ingredients:
- 1 cup orange juice
- 1/2 cup aloe vera-1/2 cup
- 1 cup celery, sliced
- 1 cup water
- handful of mint
- 1 tsp. ginger

Directions:
1. Keep your blender clean and mix orange juice with aloe vera.
2. Now add all the ingredients together and blend it for two minutes
3. That's it. Enjoy.

Nutrition:
Calories- 239
Fat-1 g
Protein- 3 g
Carbs-15 g

## 50. Swiss Chard Jazz

Preparation Time: 5 minutes
Cooking Time: 5 minutes
Servings: 2
Ingredients:
- 1 cup Swiss chard
- 1 cup blueberries
- 1 cup mixed berries
- 1 kiwi
- 2 cups spinach
- 1 cup lime juice

Directions:
1. Mix the lime juice with kiwi and spinach.
2. Now add all the ingredients together in the blender and blend it for two minutes
3. That is all. Enjoy.

Nutrition:
Calories- 239
Fat-1 g
Protein- 3 g
Carbs-15 g

## 51. Dandelion with Mango

Preparation Time: 5 minutes
Cooking Time: 5 minutes
Servings: 2
Ingredients:
- 2 cups dandelions
- 2 cups of diced mango
- 1 cup spinach
- 1 cup milk
- 1 tsp cinnamon

Directions:
1. Keep your blender clean and mix the milk and mango.
2. Now add all ingredients together and blend it for two minutes
3. That is all. Enjoy.

Nutrition:
Calories- 239
Fat-1 g
Protein- 3 g
Carbs-15 g

## 52. Sprouts Sizzles

Preparation Time: 5 minutes

Cooking Time: 5 minutes

Servings: 2

Ingredients:

- 2 cups sprouts
- 1 cup lime juice
- ½ cup spinach
- handful of mint
- 1 tsp honey

Directions:

1. First, add mints and sprouts together and blend it.
2. Now add all the ingredients and blend it for three minutes.
3. That is all. Enjoy.

Nutrition:

Calories- 239

Fat-1 g

Protein- 3 g

Carbs-15 g

## 53. Honey Green Veg

Preparation Time: 5 minutes

Cooking Time: 5 minutes

Servings: 2

Ingredients:
- spinach-2 cups
- broccoli-1 cup
- cabbage-1/2 cup
- sweet potatoes-1 piece
- honey-3 tsp
- almond milk-1 cup

Directions:

1. Mixed the milk with sweet potato and honey and blend.

2. Now add all the ingredients together and blend until thick.

3. Boil the sweet potatoes before blending. Enjoy.

Nutrition:

Calories- 239

Fat-1 g

Protein- 3 g

Carbs 15 g

## 54. Romaine Lettuce with Peach and Avocado

Preparation Time: 5 minutes

Cooking Time: 5 minutes

Servings: 2

Ingredients:

- Romaine lettuce-1 cup
- peach-1 cup
- avocado- 1 amount
- honey-2 tsp
- ginger-1 tsp
- mint-2 tsp

Directions:

1. Add all the ingredients together in the blender and blend.
2. You can use frozen fruits to make it cold.
3. That is all. Enjoy.

Nutrition:

Calories- 239

Fat-1 g

Protein- 3 g

Carbs-15 g

## 55. Pain-Reducing Pineapple Ginger

Preparation Time: 5 minutes
Cooking Time: 0 minutes
Servings: 1
Ingredients:
- 1 cup brewed and chilled green tea
- 1 cup pineapple, cut into chunks
- ½ frozen banana, sliced
- 2 tablespoons raw walnuts
- ½ teaspoon ground turmeric
- ½ teaspoon ground ginger
- 1 tablespoon ground flaxseed
- ½ to 1 cup ice
  Optional add-ins:
- 1 teaspoon bee pollen
- 1 teaspoon rosehip powder
- 1 serving hemp protein
- pinch cinnamon

Directions:
1. Combine all the ingredients and blend until smooth. Serve right away.

Nutrition:
Calories: 275;
Total Fat: 12g
Sugar: 24g
Sodium: 6mg
Carbohydrates: 40g
Fiber: 7g
Protein: 7g

## 56. Blueberry Basil Anti-Inflammatory

Preparation Time: 5 minutes
Cooking Time: 0 minutes
Servings: 1
Ingredients:
- 1 cup almond milk
- 1 cup frozen blueberries
- ½ frozen banana, sliced
- 5 to 7 large basil leaves
- 1 tablespoon tahini
- 2 tablespoons hemp seeds
- 2 cups dark leafy greens (or ½ cup frozen)
- ½ to 1 cup ice

Optional add-ins:
- ½ cup soy yogurt
- 1 serving protein powder of your choice
- ¼ cup rolled oats

Directions:
1. Combine all the ingredients and blend until smooth. Serve right away.

Nutrition:
Calories: 384;
Total Fat: 18g
Sugar: 29g
Sodium: 226mg
Carbohydrates: 49g
Fiber: 9g
Protein: 12g

## 57. Papaya Coconut Inflammation Fighter

Preparation Time: 5 minutes
Cooking Time: 0 minutes
Servings: 1
Ingredients:
- ½ cup coconut water
- ½ cup silken tofu
- 1 cup ripe papaya
- ½ cup chopped pineapple
- 2 tablespoons chia seeds
- 1 pitted Medjool date
- ½ to 1 cup ice

Optional add-ins:
- ¼ cup rolled oats
- 1 teaspoon coconut oil
- 2 tablespoons grated coconut
- 1 to 2 cups dark leafy greens

Directions:
1. Combine all the ingredients and blend until smooth. Serve right away.

Nutrition:
Calories: 271
Total Fat: 7g
Sugar: 40g
Sodium: 108mg
Carbohydrates: 52g
Fiber: 10g
Protein: 8g

## 58. Cherry Rooibos

Preparation Time: 5 minutes
Cooking Time: 0 minutes
Servings: 1
Ingredients:
- 1 cup brewed and chilled rooibos tea
- ½ cup frozen cherries
- ½ cup frozen papaya
- ¼ cup avocado
- 2 tablespoons hemp seeds
- ½ teaspoon turmeric
- ½ teaspoon ground ginger
- ½ teaspoon cinnamon
- ¼ teaspoon cayenne
- 1 pitted Medjool date
- ½ to 1 cup ice

Optional add-ins:
- 1 to 2 cups dark leafy greens (or ½ cup frozen)
- ½ frozen banana
- ½ cup frozen blueberries
- 1 teaspoon coconut oil

Directions:
1. Combine all the ingredients and blend until smooth. Serve right away.

Nutrition:
Calories: 302
Total Fat: 15g
Sugar: 29g
Sodium: 10mg
Carbohydrates: 41 g
Fiber: 8g
Protein: 8g

## 59. Coconut Carrot

Preparation Time: 5 minutes
Cooking Time: 0 minutes
Servings: 1
Ingredients:
- 1 cup unsweetened vanilla almond milk
- 1 large frozen orange, peeled and sliced
- ½ frozen banana
- ½ cup carrots, chopped
- 1 teaspoon coconut oil
- 1 tablespoon chia seeds
- 1 teaspoon turmeric powder
- pinch ground cinnamon
- pinch cayenne
- ½ teaspoon maple syrup
- ½ to 1 cup ice

Optional add-ins:
- 1 tablespoon shredded coconut
- ½ cup Greek yogurt
- ¼ cup chopped avocado

Directions:
1. Combine all the ingredients and blend until smooth. Serve right away.

Nutrition:
Calories: 288
Total Fat: 11 g
Sugar: 30g
Sodium: 220mg
Carbohydrates: 49g
Fiber: 12g
Protein: 6g

## 60. Pineapple Cherry Pain Fighter

Preparation Time: 5 minutes
Cooking Time: 0 minutes
Servings: 1
Ingredients:
- ½ cup water
- ½ cup 100% tart cherry juice
- 1 cup frozen pineapple
- 1/3 cup chopped avocado
- 1 serving hemp protein powder
- 2 cups baby spinach
- 1 teaspoon grated fresh ginger
- ½ teaspoon turmeric
- 1/8 teaspoon ground black pepper
- Stevia (optional)
- ½ to 1 cup ice

Optional add-ins:
- ½ frozen banana
- 1 tablespoon chia seeds
- ½ cup frozen cherries

Directions:
1. Combine all the ingredients and blend until smooth. Serve right away.

Nutrition:
Calories: 437
Total Fat: 13g
Sugar: 50g
Sodium: 89mg
Carbohydrates: 71 g
Fiber: 11 g
Protein: 11 g

## 61. Celery and Beet Juice

Preparation Time: 5 minutes

Cooking Time: 5 minutes

Servings: 2

Ingredients:
- 1 middle beet
- 3—4 stack of celery
- 1 carrot
- 2apples
- small piece of ginger

Directions:

1 Place everything in blender, and your bright, nutritional smoothie is ready!!!

Nutrition:

Calories: 108

Fat: 2g

Carbohydrates: 21 g

Protein: 3g

# 62. Green Almond Milk Smoothie

Preparation Time: 5 minutes

Cooking Time: 5 minutes

Servings: 2

Ingredients:

- 1.5 cups of almond milk
- 1 cup of fresh spinach
- 2 frozen bananas
- 1 spoon of honey or syrup
   Lime or lemon juice

Directions:

1. Take bananas from freezer 5 minutes before cooking.
2. Place everything in blender and pulse until finely ground.
3. The end result has to be smooth.
4. The nutritional smoothie is ready!!! Enjoy!!

Nutrition:

Calories: 108

Fat: 2g

Carbohydrates: 21 g

Protein: 3g

## 63. Green Citrus Juice

Preparation Time: 5 minutes

Cooking Time: 5 minutes

Servings: 2

Ingredients:

- 2 mandarin oranges
- large lime
- 1 lemon
- celery stalks
- kale leaves

Directions:

1 Wash all produce well.

2 Peel mandarins, lemon, and lime.

3 The nutritional smoothie is ready!!! Enjoy!!

Nutrition:

Calories: 108

Fat: 2g

Carbohydrates: 21 g

Protein: 3g

## 64. Cold Fighting Green Smoothie

Preparation Time: 5 minutes
Cooking Time: 5 minutes
Servings: 2
Ingredients:

- cup coconut water
- 1/4 cucumber
- tbsp live cultures natural yogurt
- 1/2 banana
- kiwis
- handfuls of spinach
- 1/4 tsp spirulina
- 10 drops Echinacea

Directions:
1 Peel the kiwi, wash the cucumber, and cut them into cubes.
2 Add all ingredients to the blender and mix until the ingredients are smooth.
3 Enjoy!!

Nutrition:
Calories: 108
Fat: 2g
Carbohydrates: 21 g
Protein: 3g

## 65. Fruit and Vegetable Cocktail

Preparation Time: 5 minutes

Cooking Time: 5 minutes

Servings: 2

Ingredients:

- cup unsweetened almond or coconut milk (or water)
- 1 kiwi, peeled and sliced
- 1 cup pineapple, peeled and sliced (fresh or frozen)
- 1 cucumber, peeled and sliced
- 1 cup fresh spinach
- pinch of sea salt

Directions:

1 Add all ingredients to a powerful blender and mix until smooth.

Nutrition:

Calories: 108

Fat: 2g

Carbohydrates: 21 g

Protein: 3g

## 66. Kiwi Mint Smoothie

Preparation Time: 5 minutes
Cooking Time: 5 minutes
Servings: 2
Ingredients:
- 2 kiwi
- 1/2 of green apple
- banana
- tablespoons of lemon juice
- a handful of fresh mint leaves
- cinnamon

Directions:
1. Peel all the fruits and place in the blender.
2. Add mint and pulse until smooth.
3. Add lemon juice to keep the color and a pinch of cinnamon.

Nutrition:
Calories: 108
Fat: 2g
Carbohydrates: 21 g
Protein: 3g

## 67. Avocado Smoothie

Preparation Time: 5 minutes

Cooking Time: 5 minutes

Servings: 2

Ingredients:

- 1/2 ripe avocados
- 150 ml milk of your choice (I like oat or almond)
- 40 g coconut or vanilla yogurt
- 1/2 tbsp almond butter
- tbsp honey or maple syrup
- 1 ice cube

Directions:

1 Combine ingredients in a blender and blend on high for 5 minutes.

2 Pour into a cup and enjoy.

Nutrition:

Calories: 108

Fat: 2g

Carbohydrates: 21 g

Protein: 3g

## 68. Green Lemonade

Preparation Time: 5 minutes

Cooking Time: 5 minutes

Servings: 2

Ingredients:

- 2 cucumbers
- a handful of parsley or spinach
- ½ lemon juice
- 2 cups of water
- honey

Directions:

1. Peel cucumbers and mix all the ingredients in a blender.
2. Place the drink in the fridge to cool.

Nutrition:

Calories: 108

Fat: 2g

Carbohydrates: 21 g

Protein: 3g

# 69. Sweet Spinach Detox

Preparation Time: 5 minutes

Cooking Time: 5 minutes

Servings: 2

Ingredients:
- 2 apples, peeled and cored
- lemon, peeled
- 1-inch ginger, peeled
- 30g spinach
- 2tbsp agave or honey
- 100 ml apple juice
- 100 ml water
- 6 ice cubes

Directions:

1. Gather all ingredients. Throw into your favorite blender in the order listed above.
2. Blend until desired consistency is achieved.
3. Pour into a tall glass and give your body a boost when it needs it.

Nutrition:

Calories: 108

Fat: 2g

Carbohydrates: 21 g

Protein: 3g

## 70. Celery Blueberry Smoothie

Preparation Time: 5 minutes

Cooking Time: 5 minutes

Servings: 2

Ingredients:

- 2 bananas
- 3 tablespoons of blueberries
- 1/3 of lemon juice,
- 2—3 stack of celery
- cup of water

Directions:

1. Wash and prepare ingredients.
2. Place everything in blender and pulse until finely ground. The end result has to be smooth.
3. The nutritional smoothie is ready!!! Enjoy!!

Nutrition:

Calories: 108

Fat: 2g

Carbohydrates: 21 g

Protein: 3g

# Conclusion

Smoothies are a very popular way to consume fruits and vegetables for good health. They are easy to make, convenient, and tasty. Unfortunately, people do not always make the healthiest choices. Many people use smoothies as a good excuse to drink sugary foods that contain empty calories.

However, smoothies are generally considered to be very healthy, so don't stop drinking them just yet. My tips and recipes will help you make healthier smoothies and avoid common mistakes. It will also explain how to incorporate them into your diet and why they can be important for weight loss.

It's time for you to enjoy the wonderful benefits of drinking smoothies without the drawbacks!

Smoothies have many benefits that range from nutritional to psychological. Here are some of them:

Boosts Immune System - Fruits and vegetables are packed full of vitamins, minerals, antioxidants, phytochemicals, and other beneficial nutrients that help strengthen the immune system. Smoothies are an easy way to consume them.

Natural Energy Boost - Smoothies contain fruits high in carbohydrates (sugar), so they are a great natural energy boost. The sugar is broken down by your body into glucose and released into the bloodstream as energy.

Healthy Weight Loss - Smoothies are good for weight loss because they make it easy to consume adequate calories but still maintain a calorie deficit. Many smoothies have a large quantity of protein which helps satisfy hunger and prevent overeating later in the day.

Reduce Cholesterol - Fruits and vegetables are high in fiber which helps lower bad cholesterol and keeps you healthy by lowering blood pressure. Smoothies are high in fruits which are just as good for lowering cholesterol as vegetables, but they are easier to consume because they sometimes contain a lot of liquid.

Lowers Stress - Many smoothies contain a lot of water which is good for keeping stress down. It is also an effective antidote to sugar rushes, sodas, energy drinks, and alcohol. It takes your body a while to process the fruit sugars, and it can help calm you down as a result.

Increases Stamina - A lot of smoothies contain large quantities of fruits and vegetables, which are high in vitamins and antioxidants. These help you get energy from healthy foods rather than sugars which take a while to process. They also help improve your stamina in the gym, helping you lift heavier weights without feeling fatigued.

Boosts Brain Power - Fruits have been known for centuries to be great brain food, and so are smoothies! They contain natural sugar, which your brain needs to function well.

Helps You Lose Weight - Smoothies are great for weight loss because they are healthy and high in calories. Many fruits, especially bananas, have high amounts of calories but are filling at the same time. They can help keep you satisfied instead of eating less nutrient-rich food that can leave you feeling empty and hungry later in the day.

Lowers Cholesterol - Fruits and vegetables lower bad cholesterol, which is important for helping reduce risks of heart disease. They contain extra nutrients that whole foods don't have as well as more fiber, which also helps lower cholesterol. You can also drink fruit smoothies. Sometimes, it's also very easy to include a lot of fruits in the smoothie, which can help with weight loss. Most fruits don't add up to many calories and are high in fiber and vitamins, and minerals good for your health.

Great Weight Gain - Fruits, especially those that aren't watery (bananas, avocados, kiwifruit (green), mangoes (yellow), papaya, tomatoes, etc.), will keep you satisfied longer than liquids. Because they contain calories but not an excess of them (unlike juices or sodas), you won't feel hungry later in the day.

Lightning Source UK Ltd.
Milton Keynes UK
UKHW020628060521
383207UK00003B/291